D0302343

Aromatherapy

STRESS MANAGEMENT

by Christine Westwood

Published by
Amberwood Publishing Ltd
Mulberry Court, Stour Road, Christchurch, Dorset BH23 1PS
Tel: 0202 474445

© Amberwood Publishing Ltd 1993

First Edition December 1993

All rights reserved. No part of this publication may be reproduced,
stored in a retrievable system or transmitted in any form or by any means
electronic, mechanical, photocopying, recorded or otherwise without
prior permission from the publishers Amberwood Publishing Ltd.

© Authors Copyright Christine Westwood 1993

ISBN 0-9517723-6-8

Typeset and designed by
Word Perfect, Christchurch, Dorset.

Printed in Great Britain

CONTENTS

Foreword

In my London Aromatherapy practice I treat people who come to me with a wide variety of conditions. Over the years I have come to realise that the vast majority of my clients' complaints are caused or aggravated by stress.

I practise Holistic Aromatherapy, which involves using aromatherapy essential oils to treat the entire person, rather than just addressing the symptoms. By the entire person I mean the person's physical condition; emotional state; and approach factors or events in life. The aromas I use have positive psychological and emotional effects to soothe and balance the mind. The essential oils can also help heal body systems affected by stress when they are absorbed in minute amounts via the skin.

I encourage my clients to develop life skills that will help them positively channel the stresses in their lives and discover new levels of well-being. Stressful episodes in life are inevitable, but Aromatherapy can help people use stress to their advantage by ensuring they are physically up to the challenge, mentally alert, and emotionally in balance.

During almost a decade of practising and teaching I have also developed counselling skills to augment my aromatherapy expertise. As part of their stress management programme clients examine the events, attitudes and lifestyle contributing to their stress and causing their symptoms. If they are not happy with aspects of their lifestyle I encourage them to explore possibilities for change and to use Aromatherapy to maintain their health.

I am writing this book to share the benefit of my experience so readers can examine the nature of stress in their lives and manage their stress positively by the use of essential oils.

My thanks go to my friends, colleagues, and family who encouraged me to write this sequel to my first book, *Aromatherapy – A Guide for Home Use*.

Special thanks are due to Sabre Gilmartin, who edited this book.

Christine Westwood MIFA, TDHA

1 | What is Stress?

Stress is one of the biggest influences in our lives today: from decision making executives; to isolated housewives; to children confronted by playground bullies. Our reactions to stress and the resulting adaptations we make to our lifestyles can make all the difference to our health and happiness. So let's look at some of the concepts involved before exploring how Aromatherapy can help.

Recent widespread recognition and focus on the importance of stress might lead us to believe that stress is a relatively new phenomenon caused by faster travel, global business or computerisation. This is not so by any means. People for many centuries have had to deal with stressed lifestyles. What may be new today are some ways of looking at and dealing with issues related to stress and the broad popularity of Stress Management Training.

The medical profession is placing increasing emphasis on studying stress and its effects. This is partly related to greater popular interest, but is mainly because stress has now been linked as a major causative factor in such serious conditions as coronary heart disease, cancer, chronic digestive disorders and late onset diabetes.

Stress itself is an inevitable part of life. Dr. Hans Selye, an internationally recognised authority on the subject, has written: Stress can be avoided only by dying. Most of the potential stressors or opportunities we meet every day we handle in our stride. Our positive response to these events provides interest, challenge and excitement to our lives. Unresolved stressful situations, however, built up over time, can cause us problems.

❀ *Flight or Fight*
Various writers and experts have suggested different definitions for stress. These range from looking at stress in a totally negative light to describing it as a necessary part of our lives upon which we can thrive.

Flight or fight is a widely accepted interpretation of the response to stress that was first described earlier this century by Walter B Cannon. Cannon was an American Nobel Prize winning physiologist who studied and described the body's spontaneous reactions to stressors. The response stimulates our body's production of hormones including adrenaline. These hormones prompt a number of alert responses including increased

5

pupil dilation, heightened muscle tension, faster heart rate, and raised blood pressure. Our liver then converts stored glycogen to glucose and releases it into the blood stream. At the same time our digestion is inhibited because the blood it would require is diverted to our muscles and brain. These physical reactions to stressors prepare us either to run away from the situation (flight), or to confront the situation (fight), therefore they are called the flight or fight response.

Frequently society's demands don't let us respond to the situation by either fighting or running away! There are often occasions when for one reason or another we mask our reactions. Our bodies then remain in a state of stress, which can become health-threatening. Stomach ulcers are one example of a physical outcome that can result if the body is subjected to repeated or prolonged stress. These ulcers are lesions caused when the body's protective secretions, that normally neutralise stomach acid, are inhibited by stress.

❀ *Adaptation*
The General Adaptation Syndrome is Dr. Hans Selye's name for his description of the physical stress response. Selye's writings, combined with the earlier work by Cannon, help us to understand the effects of prolonged stress on the body. Selye divides the stress response into three phases: The Alarm Response, Adaptation, and Exhaustion.

The Alarm Response is like the flight or fight preparation by the body that was previously described by Cannon. During this initial phase we become alert and ready for action. In exceptional cases our physical resistance to the stressor may become weakened, for example as a consequence of severe burns, shock or extremes of temperature.

In Selye's second phase, Adaptation, our bodies physically adjust to a stressful situation when acute signs of the initial alarm reaction have subsided and we are in a recovery state. If we encounter another stressor at this stage, a new acute reaction occurs before our body can completely restore balance.

If this continues, Exhaustion, Selye's third stage, may result because our body doesn't have a chance to regain equilibrium and settle down to normal functioning before each flight or fight response takes over.

Most of us have experienced one thing after another going wrong, stressing us to the point where even the slightest negative thing makes us want to weep or scream. This is an example of the body going through The General Adaptation Syndrome and having new stressors repeatedly occurring before previous ones are resolved. The result of this physiological and emotional roller coaster is what we commonly call a "high stress level".

❀ Positive Stress

Stressors, can however, be positive as well as negative. Excitement such as news of a major win on the pools provokes the same body reactions as a sudden fright. When we take part in thrill-seeking activities like amusement park rides, bungee jumping or speedboat racing, we are triggering our stress responses on purpose. It's the rush of adrenaline that gives us that feeling of exhilaration after which the stress is quickly released. Here we experience and enjoy our flight or fight response as excitement.

Just as the stress response isn't always provoked by something negative the effect of stress need not always be negative. The increased resources we experience when we are stressed can galvanise us into action, enabling us to rise to the occasion in difficult circumstances. In that case, instead of building exhaustingly high stress levels, we get a satisfying feeling of elation from our accomplishment and a sense of physical well-being.

The way people react to stress can range from lack of motivation, depression and anxiety to the opposite extreme of a continued frenzy of over-achievement. Neither extreme is healthy. People's needs in life differ. For some people having too few stimuli can trigger a stress response. These people may thrive on continual new challenge and a lifestyle that is like an ongoing Outward Bound course. Other people require a quiet lifestyle and don't need much stimulation.

Whatever your needs and expectations from life, Aromatherapy can help you control your physical and emotional stress responses so you can achieve and maintain a healthy balance. By using essential oils and Aromatherapy techniques as part of a programme of positive stress management, you can turn stressors into opportunities to heighten your achievements while keeping your physical and emotional systems in balance.

2 | Positive Stress Management

Many people would approach stress management with the aim of eliminating all the effects of stress in their lives. On the contrary, the goal of positive stress management is to harness and control the effects of stress to enhance physical and mental power.

Positive Stress Management involves recognising the existence and qualitative level of stress and then formulating and following a plan of action.

❀ Recognising Stress
Often before you can recognise and deal with the root cause of a stress-related condition, you need to treat the symptoms of stress. You might initially be prompted to do something about stress because of a symptom such as a headache. If you have a stress-induced headache, it indicates you are out of balance. Aromatherapy can help you regain a state of equilibrium. When your balance is restored, and you are in a more positive frame of mind, you can step back and look at your previous stressed state. Then you are in a stronger position and can take hold of the situation to make your stresses work for you.

❀ Formulating Your Aroma Action Plan
Stress management planning normally happens on two levels, sub-conscious and conscious. On the sub-conscious level your body physically responds to stress and will respond to aromas without your needing to think about it. On a conscious level, you may decide to formulate a plan of action and choose how you will respond. Essential oils can help when you are deciding your approach to a situation because they restore mental balance, encouraging a relaxed yet alert state of mind.

❀ Making Your Stresses Work for You
The often used expression – Turning a negative into a positive – is relevant to positive stress management. We have looked at the ways our bodies prepare for action in response to stressors. You can use a stress-induced heightened physical state to rise above your normal level of achievement. The trick is learning how to do it. Some people have a natural flair for tapping their resources and coming out ahead; others learn; and some never master it at all. We've all met people who say they

work more effectively under stress or with deadlines. Similarly we probably know people who were totally unaware of their ability until they were faced with a disastrous or chaotic situation and had to take charge. The stress in the situation actually enabled the person to get in touch with their hidden talents.

You can use your stressors as an opportunity to focus your mind and creatively work towards a solution. When you are at the positive height of your stress response you can also be at your most creative. That's when you can harness your energy to deal effectively with a challenge. If you continually evaluate and plan the way you're dealing with situations, you can maximise both your effectiveness and your sense of well-being. You will also be more able to cope with unexpected or acute stresses as well as a generally stressful lifestyle pattern. You will then be dealing with potential stressors before they have a chance to become chronic patterns.

✣ Following Your Aroma Action Plan
Including Aromatherapy as a major feature of your stress management plan will help you achieve and maintain the physical and mental condition you need to meet new stresses and continue to deal effectively with current stress levels. Aromatherapy methods of using the essential oils include:

• Massage with essential oils
• Aromatherapy baths
• Compresses
• Scalp treatments
• Room fragrancers
• Inhalation
• Perfume blends

Consult the indexes in this book to help you select the oils and methods that best suit your circumstances.

3 | Stress Quiz

Tick the boxes for all questions that apply to you.

Physical
1. Do you feel you sleep too much or too little? ☐
2   Do you have difficulty sitting still and relaxing? ☐
3. Do you suffer neck or back pain from tense or stiff muscles? ☐

Mental
4. Are you constantly irritable or easily angered? ☐
5. Do you find it difficult to concentrate? ☐
6. Are you often forgetful? ☐

Emotional
7. Do you feel as if everything is piling up on top of you? ☐
8. Do you feel anxious or uneasy a lot of the time? ☐
9. Do you sometimes feel keyed up, over excited, or hyperactive? ☐

Lifestyle
10. Are you generally unhappy with your lifestyle? ☐
11. Do you fail to follow your chosen values? ☐
12. Have you developed the habit of drinking, eating or smoking excessively? ☐

Personal
13. Are you unable to pace yourself to allow periods of re-energising? ☐
14. Do you fail to reward yourself for your successes? ☐
15. Do you find "empty time" lonely and stressful? ☐

Relationships
16. Do you find it difficult to talk to others? ☐
17. Do you have difficulty with relationships - even with those you love the most? ☐
18. Do you tend to be withdrawn? ☐

Surroundings
19. Do you live or work in an area with a high noise level? ☐
20. Do you suffer from environmental stress? ☐
21. Do your surroundings conflict with your desired lifestyle? ☐

❁ Scoring

Give yourself one point for each box ticked. Take note whether there are one or more categories where you have a higher concentration of ticks and resolve to particularly concentrate on those areas when formulating a self-help Aromatherapy stress management plan. Use the Indexes and Methods Section of this book to choose your essential oils and method of application.

Score	Analysis and Recommendations
17-21	A complete lifestyle review is indicated including regular Aromatherapy sessions and use of essential oils.
12-16	You probably have a fairly high stress level for which an Aromatherapy stress management plan would be advised. You may want to discuss it with a supportive partner or friend who can help you formulate and carry it out.
7-11	There may be a few specific areas in your life that you could explore and address using this book for guidance.
1-6	Life would be boring without some stress but congratulations for generally taking care of yourself. Focus on using essential oils to help with the stress areas you identified and to maintain an acceptable stress level.

❁ Life Skills to Complement Aromatherapy

There are other actions you may want to take to complement your Aromatherapy stress management plan. You might already have some ideas or you could begin by reviewing this list of suggestions and goals and choose ones you feel would enhance your life and which appeal to you.
• Reflection and review of your lifestyle.
• Relaxation & meditation or focusing.
• Physical activity e.g. taking a walk or playing a sport.
• Healthy eating.
• Hobbies and recreation.
• Self-esteem and assertiveness.
• Review your home environment and remove clutter.
• Time management.
• Financial planning and management.
• Developing communication and listening skills.
• Relationships and socialising.
• Goal setting.

❁ Actions

• List your stressors (stress indicators).
• Set aside time for yourself.

- Locate interesting books to help carry out your self-help programme. (See Helpful Books Section).
- Follow an Adult Education Course at your local college to gain or enhance your skills and knowledge in these areas. Courses are generally offered from beginner to advanced levels.
- Local libraries have lists of special interest groups. With one of these groups you can start a new hobby or rekindle an old one. This is a good way of meeting people with similar interests.
- In some areas there are child care support groups where parents take it in turn to mind children so they can have time for themselves. Other groups or classes welcome family participation.

4 | Stressors and Indicated Aromas Chart

YOURSELF

Stressor	Objectives	Essential Oil
Boredom	Stimulate Interest	Jasmine, Rosemary
Fear of Intimacy	Courage	Frankincense
Feeling Rejected	Openness	Frankincense, Jasmine, Rose
Disease, Injury	Treatment & Essential Oils★	See index for oils
Insomnia	Relaxation	Lavender
Jet Lag	Stimulation	Peppermint, Rosemary
Lack of Assertiveness	Confidence	Frankincense
	Self-Esteem	Sandalwood
Over-Analytical	Trust	Ylang Ylang
Poor Time Management	Relaxation	Lavender
	Focus	Grapefruit
	Memory Stimulant	Rosemary
Workaholism	Balance	Geranium
Worry	Faith	Chamomile

YOUR RELATIONSHIPS

Bereavement	Heal Grief	Rose
Divorce or Separation	Acceptance & Letting Go	Rose
Family Problems	Objectivity & Clarity	Rosemary
Peer Pressure	Inner Strength	Frankincense
Unemployment	Positivity	Bergamot, Cajeput

YOUR SURROUNDINGS

Allergens	Strengthen Immune System	Lavender
Fear of Future	Empowerment & Acceptance	Neroli
Financial Change:	Acceptance	Neroli
Worse/Better	Action Planning	Basil, Rosemary
Insecurity re Home/		
Business	Steadiness	Frankincense
Pollution	Cleansing	Rose
Society's Expectations	True to Self	Frankincense

★This chart gives examples of stressors with suggested objectives for change and associated essential oils. It is by no means intended as a comprehensive list of stressors. You could use this chart to help you begin to review your own lifestyle and circumstances to identify your stressors along with any changes you would like to make. You can then use this with the other charts in this book to choose your own essential oils.

5 | Physical & Emotional Stress Responses

The Fight or Flight Syndrome and the Adaptation Response discussed in the previous chapter concern our body's ways of responding to and dealing with stress. Now we will take a more detailed look at individual body systems to help us recognise the physical and emotional symptoms caused by stress. Our mental and emotional responses to events affect our physical well-being. The better we understand the body's processes, the more able we are to react positively to stress and avoid its negative effects.

❀ *The Skin*
The skin is our body's largest eliminative organ. It releases toxins through perspiration and continuous shedding of dead skin layers. An effect of stress on the skin is to increase our toxin levels. The higher toxin levels trigger hormonal imbalances. The visible effects of stress upon the skin take various forms, including:
• Acne
• Blemishes, spots and premature ageing of the skin
• Eczema
• Furrowed forehead lines
• Pallor due to muscular tension withdrawing blood from the skin's surface – hence the expression "going white with fright"
• Psoriasis
• Sagging skin in the jaw area
• Skin diseases
  Aromatherapy is a great aid to stress-related skin problems since our skin absorbs minute amounts of the essential oils from bathing or massage which help restore physical and emotional balance.

❀ *Digestive and Eliminative System*
When we are stressed, our digestive system shuts down. Our mouths become dry and secretion of stomach-juices is inhibited. If we eat while we are under stress, food is not properly digested. As the improperly digested food moves through the colon imbalanced nutrients are absorbed into the bloodstream. As a result our intestines and bowels can become irritated and, in the long term, stress can lead to persistent stomach ache, peptic ulcers, colitis or irritable bowel syndrome. If you

have any of these problems you should seek medical help and a qualified Aromatherapy practitioner.

Using essential oils for the digestive and eliminative system can promote and maintain a healthy digestive system. Aromatherapy can support conventional medical treatment for stress-related digestive disorders and help to prevent these conditions from occurring. If you are feeling stressed when you need to eat, try limiting yourself to light meals of easily digestible food and using relaxation techniques combined with essential oils. In the United Kingdom, Aromatherapy practice does not advocate oral use of essential oils. External application permits absorption over a period of several hours and has been found to be more appropriate.

✤ *Respiratory and Cardiovascular Systems*

Shortness of breath due to muscles tightening is an effect of stress on our respiratory system. Prolonged shallow breathing, in turn, affects our cardiovascular system, which includes the heart, arteries and veins. When we consistently breath shallowly our body is not able to sufficiently purify the blood. Toxins and excessive hormones therefore remain in the bloodstream. The processes of the respiratory and cardiovascular systems are very closely linked.

The respiratory system consists of the nose, throat and lungs. There are small sacs in the lungs, called alveoli, in which oxygen enters the bloodstream and impurities like carbon dioxide are removed. The respiratory system is affected by environmental stressors and by our emotional state. Environmental stressors acting on the respiratory system include air pollutants, poor air conditioning systems, central heating, smoking, allergens and electronic stress from computer emissions. All of this affects our breathing and therefore our health.

Breathing fully and deeply promotes healing and gives us a glow of vitality and a sense of well-being. Shallower breathing caused by stress leads to a decrease in our oxygen supply, which can create a sense of panic. Aromatherapy can help us combat shallow breathing and panic by promoting mental relaxation and a state of concentration similar to that achieved by meditation. Certain essential oils have a direct link with the respiratory system and encourage deep full breathing leading to relaxation. This promotes mental and emotional well-being as well as contributing to the optimal functioning of our physical systems. When we are relaxed, our heart and respiration rates slow down and our skin temperature increases. Relaxation also enhances our ability to focus so that we can concentrate on improving our quality of life and our commitment to personal and professional goals. This can also have a positive effect on stress-related physical conditions including asthma, high blood pressure and high serum cholesterol levels.

Stress and Respiratory Disease – Experiments have shown that people are more prone to upper respiratory disease when they are undergoing significant and stressful life events. One study of forty, first-year medical students showed that when their activities were curtailed due to illness, it was primarily during exam periods. Another study showed that people reported increased stress three to four days before they came down with upper respiratory infections. This correlates with the 24-72 hour incubation period of many common cold viruses. Stress lowers our immune systems and can thus make us more predisposed to disease.

Aromatherapy can be an aid to disease prevention. Essential oils absorbed by inhalation or through the skin can soothe respiratory conditions and help release anxiety. As the essential oils are inhaled, they promote increased bronchial mucus which aids the healing process for many types of respiratory infection. Essential oils used in fragrancers are particularly effective at killing airborne bacteria that are linked with infections.

❀ Immune System

The immune system is our body's defence against infection; it includes the lymph system and associated organs. When we are under sustained or major stress, the immune system can be weakened, making us more susceptible to infections.

The body, aided by an efficiently operating immune system, has many defences against toxins and disease. Sneezing and coughing are a first line defence against the entry of toxins into our bodies. The mucous linings of the ear, nose and throat passages have tiny cilia which sift out irritants like bacteria, viruses and allergens. When we do become ill, and react with a fever, our metabolic rate and blood and lymph circulation increase to speed up removal of the toxins that made us ill. Sweating also facilitates faster elimination of toxins through the skin.

Our mental and emotional state can affect efficient operation of our immune system. American scientists observing severely ill patients have discovered that regular viewing of humorous videos produced measurable health improvement and in some cases has even promoted recovery. Laughter can really be a great healer.

Essential oils can be a powerful support for the immune system in helping prevent infection. The majority of oils have anti-bacterial properties and, in addition, some have either anti-viral or anti-fungal properties. Tea tree oil in particular has all three.

❀ Nervous, Hormonal and Reproductive Systems

Our stress response starts in the nervous system, which links the brain, the spine and the nerves. Our brain signals the hormonal system, which releases hormones, including adrenaline, into the bloodstream to help our body respond to the stressor. The endocrine glands, which include the adrenal, pituitary and thyroid glands, are involved in this response.

As our body produces adrenaline, we experience, according to the way we perceive it, either anxiety or excitement. The effects of unresolved stress on the nervous and hormonal systems can lead to a wide range of mental and emotional imbalances and can lay a foundation for disease. This may lead to hyperactivity, nervousness and, if prolonged, to exhaustion.

The endocrine system also produces hormones called endorphins which work to counteract negative effects of stress by promoting pleasurable thoughts and feelings. Aromatherapy can encourage our bodies to release endorphins by stimulating the Limbic System, located in the brain, which in turn stimulates the endocrine system.

The reproductive system is also influenced by stress. Women may find that stress affects their menstrual cycle. Oestrogen and progesterone levels may become unbalanced. Stress can contribute to gynaecological problems associated with pre-menstrual syndrome, childbirth or menopause. Male reproductive systems can also be adversely affected by stress and in severe cases this can even lead to impotence.

Hormonal imbalances can be helped by using certain essential oils which have properties similar to the body's reproductive hormones. Conditions like menstrual pain are often exacerbated by lack of exercise, bad nutrition and disturbed sleep. When we start using essential oils we typically begin to experience improved sleep patterns which make us feel better and improve our frame of mind. Good quality sleep aids repair and renewal of our body. Our posture and outlook become more positive and we generally have a greater sense of well-being.

❀ *Muscular and Skeletal Systems*
As part of the stress reaction, our muscles tense up ready for action. If we experience prolonged fear or are habitually anxious, our muscles become fixed in a tense position. As a result of continued stress, our muscles may lose their suppleness and our posture may be adversely affected, becoming rigid or collapsed. This may be painful and affect proper working of our major organs.

When our muscles are contracting due to stress they are working and they need nourishment. Our blood flow slows down, though, because the blood is unable to flow freely through the contracted muscle tissue. This retards nourishment and causes toxins, which are a by-product of the work, to build up. We can experience this as inflammation or pain or both. This pain stimulates our body to release hormones which can increase blood pressure and cause inflammation in the skin, joints and mucous membranes. This has been associated with conditions such as arthritis, pruritis, dermatitis and asthma. Persistent or chronic muscle tension and resulting over-production of hormones can deplete the immune system and lower our resistance to infections.

The skeletal system has over a thousand muscles which are always in some degree of tension or relaxation. These muscles support the skeleton and help us move. The muscles also hold our major organs in the right positions. Usually we are unaware of the tension level in individual muscle groups but sometimes it can be useful to make ourselves consciously aware of the level of tension. Through this awareness and by focusing on letting go, we can begin to release our tension and prevent a further build up of tension. A good way of doing this is to make ourselves aware of each group of muscles in the body in turn tensing and releasing them while maintaining awareness of the depth of our breathing. When our breathing is too shallow, our muscles don't receive the optimum level of oxygen and we feel tired.

❀ Suggested Routine for Releasing Muscular Tension

These simple exercises are best performed several times a day at a regular time or when you have a few minutes free. Then when stressful or potentially stressful situations arise, you already have a way of releasing stress.

Hand and Forearm	Make a tight fist, hold for a few seconds and release.
Upper Arm	Press elbow and forearm down against the surface of a table or chair, hold and release.
Forehead	Raise eyebrows as far as possible, hold and let go.
Upper Cheeks and Nose	Scrunch eyes and wriggle nose, then release.
Chest and Shoulders	Pull shoulders up as far as you can toward the ears, let go, then pull shoulder blades together and release.
Abdomen	Hold stomach out then pull it in and release.

Do this in conjunction with regular Aromatherapy baths and/or massage.

Hand and foot massage is beneficial for the muscular and skeletal systems and is something we can do ourselves. Both the hands and feet contain acupressure points which can influence the whole body.

Some essential oils promote an analgesic effect which can ease swollen joints, rheumatism or stiff muscles. Oils such as Juniper, Rosemary and Black Pepper have a rubefacient, or warming, effect which improves blood flow to the muscles. They can make your skin feel warm and give you a pink glow.

❀ Mind, Emotions and Sense of Smell

The effect of Aromatherapy on the mind is a fascinating subject. Throughout history aromatic oils such as Sandalwood have been used to influence our emotions and state of mind. Sandalwood is a key ingredient of incense, which is used to calm and focus the mind.

We first inhale aromas through our nose which sends messages interpreting the aroma to the brain. There is also a touch sensitive system located in the nose, called the trigeminal system, which reacts to pungent substances like ammonia, acetone and carbon dioxide and triggers us to turn our heads and back away in response to those substances. It is the limbic system in the brain that receives and responds to aroma stimuli. The limbic system also forms the root of our mental and emotional responses so that aromas can profoundly effect our mental state and emotional health.

The acuteness of our sense of smell can change during the course of our lives or temporarily due to illness. Babies spontaneously respond to aromas simply as stimuli without classifying them as good or bad, harmful or benign. They may, in fact, need to be guided away from harmful substances. Young people tend to be experimental with smells as they are with everything else in their lives. As adults we are likely to have already categorised aromas into likes and dislikes. Older people sometimes suffer a lessening of their sense of smell. Because over 80% of our ability to taste is related to our sense of smell, loss of ability to smell is accompanied by loss of ability to distinguish tastes. This can lead to reduction of appetite and enjoyment of meals. The deprivation of stimuli which accompanies reduced sense of smell may bring with it with feelings of depression.

Sometimes we have a temporary loss of smell because we have a cold or have been in an accident. When we have a cold, the reduced sense of smell can actually play a part in our recovery. It lessens our interest in food and causes us to eat less. Our body resources are therefore freer to fight the infection rather than working on digestion. This is only true for part of the illness cycle. As we get better, our appetite returns because we need nourishment to complete our healing.

Our mind and emotions are constantly affected by our reactions to odour stimuli from the environment. By using Aromatherapy essential oils we have a greater degree of control over our aroma stimuli to bring about the effects and balance we desire.

The Stress Response Index near the end of this book gives specific information on the use of essential oils for our mental and emotional well-being.

❈ Holistic Stress Management with Aromatherapy

We've looked at individual body systems to help us understand some of the physical and mental effects of stress reactions. Over and above the importance of treating individual symptoms, scientific observation and research has shown an holistic approach to be the best way of dealing with stress. That means working with the whole person. If you have a symptom like nausea, headaches or eczema, first you will want to deal with your physical condition. (See the Physical Conditions Index).

Your symptoms may be the result of factors affecting you in your relationships, your homelife or your work. Making yourself consciously aware of these stressful aspects of life and listing them can be therapeutic in itself. It can help you put things into perspective and help you decide what you want to do about them. Not acknowledging and dealing with things that are causing us stress can lead to serious harm both physically and mentally. For that reason an holistic Aromatherapist tries to obtain as much information about a patient as possible when working with them on a course of therapy.

After examining your lifestyle and stresses you will become more aware of how you personally respond to the stressors in your life. You can then use the Stress Response Index at the back of this book to select essential oils to address the root causes in connection with the Physical Conditions Index.

6 | Aromatherapy Methods for Stress

There are several methods of using Aromatherapy essential oils, all of which are very enjoyable and provide a basis for ongoing good health:

❀ *Massage*

Massage has been found to be the most effective way of using essential oils. The balancing properties of the essential oils encourage the desired response using small amounts. Varying from the suggested strength, however, can actually result in the opposite of the intended result. For example, Lavender essential oil is relaxing but in too great a strength it is stimulating Similarly, a small amount of Peppermint essential oil is stimulating but used in larger quantities produces the opposite – a soporific effect.

A full Aromatherapy massage is wonderful for relieving and healing stress related conditions. For that, it is best to go to a trained holistic Aromatherapist. However, you can give yourself or a friend a hand or foot massage or, if you want to be more adventurous, you can take a basic Aromatherapy course which will teach you to give a good back massage. Back massage is very helpful because shoulders and backs often give us the first signals that we are "under stress".

METHOD
• Choose a base oil like sweet almond oil in which to blend the essential oils.
• Fill a 10 millilitre bottle with the base oil. (The capacity is usually found on the bottom of brown glass bottles.)
• Choose the essential oils for your blend using the indexes and advice in this book. You might choose for example, a mix of Lavender for relaxation; Sandalwood to release tension in the throat area; and Bergamot to uplift.
• Mix the blend:
To get the maximum number of drops of essential oil divide the number of millilitres in the bottle by two. For a 10 millilitre bottle this means the maximum is 5 drops of essential oil, though you can use fewer than 5 for a more subtle blend.

Suggested proportions of the above would be:

Sandalwood	1 drop
Bergamot	2 drops
Lavender	1 drop

This totals 4 drops, and is still under the suggested maximum for a 10 millilitre bottle.

✿ Bathing

At the Start of the Day – Use the essential oils to stimulate your mind and protect your body for the day ahead. Examples of these are Rosemary which will stimulate the mind and Lavender for protection of the immune system. See the indexes for more comprehensive information to make your own choice.

At the End of the Day – Choose oils like Geranium, Lavender or Clary Sage which will help you to unwind and relax.

METHOD
• Run a bath which is not so hot as to cause the oils to evaporate.
• Add 3-5 drops of essential oil.
• Agitate the water.
• Soak in the bath and relax for 10-15 minutes.
• Gently dry yourself to allow maximum absorption of the oils.

✿ Compress

"Soothing a troubled brow' – This well-known expression refers to an important location – the brow or forehead. Stroking the brow or holding your head in your hands links into the pressure points for emotional release located in the forehead. Thus by stroking the brow or placing a compress with essential oils on it, the tension is eased. The back of the neck or aching limbs also respond well to compresses.

METHOD
• Prepare the blend as for massage.
• Follow first-aid procedures to make the compress and to choose the appropriate water temperature.
• Add one to two drops of essential oil to a small bowl of water.
• Gently lay the compress on the water.
• Place the compress on the affected area.

✿ Scalp Treatment

A blend can be used for scalp massage, which is an excellent way of releasing tension and for treating dandruff.

METHOD
- Massage an essential oil blend well into the scalp and leave it on for half an hour. It is best to do this in the bath or sauna.
- Apply shampoo without using any water at this point (the oils do not mix with water).
- Once the hair is coated you can proceed with your normal hair–washing routine, including rinsing thoroughly with water.
- You can add a couple of drops of essential oil to the final rinse.

❀ *Room Fragrancer*

You can use essential oils with a fragrancer to create a special atmosphere. Rosemary is stimulating. Lavender is relaxing. Lemongrass and citrus oils like Orange, Lemon or Bergamot are refreshing after a warm summer day. Spicy oils such as Cinnamon and Clove in a blend with Orange or Rosewood are particularly welcoming in the Autumn and Winter.

As we inhale the fragrance we are also protected from airborne bacteria. This minimises infections from colds and flu.

METHODS
1. Fragrancer
- Choose one with a deep well.
- Fill it three-quarters full with water.
- Add up to 5 drops of essential oil.
- Light a night light candle which will burn for up to 5 hours.
- If you choose a fragrancer with a cut-out pattern you can enjoy a pleasing reflection on the wall or ceiling which enhances the relaxing effect.
  N.B. Do not leave the night light unattended and extinguish it at the end of use.
2. Vaporiser Ring – This is a ceramic ring which fits over a light bulb and has a channel in which you pour the essential oil.
- Place the ring on a cool light bulb.
- Add up to 5 drops of essential oil and turn the light on.
3. Dish – You can put a few drops of essential oil in a saucer of water and place it on the radiator.

❀ *Inhalation*

Inhalation is good for relieving congestion, easing catarrh and soothing the respiratory tract.

METHOD
- Pour two pints of boiling water into a bowl.
- Add 10 drops of an essential oil indicated for the chest like Eucalyptus, Camphor or Thyme; or a blend of these essential oils.
- Agitate the water.

- Put a towel over your head. Close your eyes and inhale the vapours for a few minutes at a time for up to ten minutes or as long as is comfortable.
- Repeat this several times a day as desired.
- A facial steamer with 5 drops of essential oil may be used instead of the bowl.

Perfume

Use a blend of the essential oils you enjoy and dab it on the inside of the wrist and behind the ear. (Prepare the blend as for massage). Neroli included in a blend acts as a good stress protector.

You can also inhale the essential oils by putting one to two drops of essential oil on a handkerchief or tissue, inhaling as required. You could, for example, use Peppermint for travel sickness or Lavender for tension.

7 | Case Histories

I am including the following case histories with clients' permission, although names and details have been changed to preserve anonymity. These are based on sessions with my clients and give specific illustrations of how Aromatherapy may be used for stress management. These profiles provide examples only and do not presume to cover all types of situations and lifestyles.

❧ Marianne

Marianne, a 45-year-old divorcée, consulted me saying she was suffering from stress, tension, exhaustion and chronic indigestion. She separated from her husband five years ago. She says she has now almost come to terms with her situation, and has just begun a new relationship.

To support herself and four children she set up a small business which is now doing well. She describes herself as being hyperactive and says she worries a lot about her business and her children especially as her business takes her away from home. She devotes no time to herself. Although she prepares regular meals for the children, she eats irregularly, between her other activities.

Attitude to Life and Self-Understanding – Marianne has worked hard to build a firm base. However, she is not enjoying the benefits of her hard work because she has been living in the past. If she takes time to review her current lifestyle, keeping in mind her commitments, she could plan time for herself to begin to relax and enjoy what she has accomplished. Marianne could do herself a lot of good by acknowledging her achievements and realising that loving and nurturing herself will enable her to accomplish even more if she wishes. she can then explore what she wants for her family and in her new relationship.

SELF-HELP PROGRAMME AND LIFESTYLE BALANCE
• Regular Aromatherapy baths.
• Weekly Aromatherapy massage.
• Developing time management and business delegation skills. This would give more time for herself and her children.
• Learning relaxation techniques and taking time to relax.
• Organising regular meals for herself.
• Developing her social life.

• Setting support systems in place and enlisting help from the family.
• Having a live-in au-pair thus creating free time for hobbies or interests which would provide social contact.

SUGGESTED ESSENTIAL OILS TO CHOOSE FROM FOR HER BLEND
Mental & Emotional Level:

> Clary Sage to uplift her.
> Camomile to soothe her hyperactivity.
> Rose to release lingering grief from the divorce.
> Sandalwood to bring her worries into perspective.
> Melissa to enhance her femininity.

Physical Level:

> Fennel for her digestive system.
> Neroli to balance her overworked adrenal system.
> Lavender for relaxation.

Suggested Blend:

Clary Sage	1
Neroli	1
Lavender	2

4 drops in a 10 ml. base for massage or added to bath water.

Once she experiences relaxation from Aromatherapy massage with Lavender, and her adrenal system is in balance after using Neroli, her other symptoms may disappear. If not she can continue therapy with a blend from the other suggested essential oils.

❀ *Laura*

Laura is 28 and single. She suffers from frequent migraines and chronic backache. she works in an office where she spends hours each day in front of a computer screen. Laura is a perfectionist who considers herself a failure because she didn't go to university. She gets frustrated when she makes mistakes and often takes on more than her share of work having to stay late at the office to complete it. Both Laura's parents are ill and she spends her weekends looking after them. That is when she gets most of her migraines.

Attitude to Life and Self-Understanding – Laura would do well to explore her perfectionist, driven approach to life and to find ways to take care of herself. She can then begin to develop a more positive attitude about herself and her current achievements. Does Laura really want to go to university? If so, how will she go about it? If not, is this a past ambition which is no longer relevant to her life? She could also look at the reasons why she takes so much on herself and what she could do to take care of herself

SELF-HELP PROGRAMME AND LIFESTYLE BALANCE
- Using relaxation and self-help Aromatherapy to nurture herself.
- Developing time management and assertiveness skills which will enable her to organise her workload and say no when appropriate.
- Using an ioniser and computer screen as protection from electronic stress.
- Taking regular screen breaks.
- Researching opportunities for university or other further education courses.
- Finding additional or alternative ways of getting her parents the help and support they need, possibly by enlisting other family members.
- Practising enjoyable exercise, including taking time out for relaxation with friends.

SUGGESTED ESSENTIAL OILS
Mental & Emotional Level:

Melissa for its nurturing effect and to soothe the mind.

Ylang Ylang for resentment about her circumstances and to soften her tendency to self-criticism.

Rose to open her up to the present.

Frankincense for self-confidence and self-worth.

Physical Level:

Lavender used in massage for backache.

Neroli and Orange for electronic stress.

Marjoram for deep relaxation.

Suggested Blend:

Frankincense	1
Neroli	2
Marjoram	1
	4 drops

Taking time for herself, initially by taking Aromatherapy baths, will promote relaxation whilst Frankincense will encourage self-confidence giving her the boost she needs to examine her situation and make choices for herself.

❦ *Stephen*

Stephen is a 55-year-old married man who has a drinking problem and suffers from eczema. He was unexpectedly made redundant two years ago and has been unable to find work since. He is suffering difficulties in his relationships with his wife and their youngest son, who is still at home. He is smoking more and goes to the pub by himself most lunch times and evenings.

Attitude to Life and Self-Understanding – Stephen could use his present situation to step back and review his life, acknowledging his skills and capabilities and "brainstorming" new ways of employing them. He could also consider the possibility of learning new skills. He needs to realise that self-worth is not only dependent on his professional role or work situation.

SELF–HELP PROGRAMME AND LIFESTYLE BALANCE
• Regular aromatherapy sessions and home use of essential oils.
• Seeking professional help to reduce drinking.
• Finding a positive support group instead of the pub.
• Looking for ways to improve family relationships.
• Seeking out charities or other organisations where he could put his time and skills to constructive use.
• Developing a plan of action.
• Cultivating positive activities and interests.
• Taking regular exercise appropriate to his physical condition.
• Learning about and practising healthy nutrition.

SUGGESTED ESSENTIAL OILS
Mental & Emotional Level:

        Clary Sage for addictive patterns.
        Ylang Ylang to release resentment.
        Rose to release the past.
        Jasmine to help open out to new possibilities.
Physical Level:
        Geranium for skin problems.
        Lavender for skin and immune system.
        Juniper for its cleansing properties.
Suggested Blend:

Juniper	1
Lavender	2
Ylang Ylang	1

$\overline{}$
4 drops

    Stephen is going through a period of adjusting to the loss of his job and the resultant changes in his life. He needs support to channel his energies in a more positive way to explore new possibilities whilst accepting his current situation.

❀ *Alan*
Alan is a student and active sportsman whose studies are going well, although he gets tired preparing for major exams. Alan loves running and wants to enter a cross-country race in two months.
    Attitude to Life and Self-Understanding – Alan's attitude is already very positive and should help him achieve his immediate goals of successfully

completing his studies and doing well in the race. Alan could learn more about good nutrition and use essential oils to keep him in tip-top condition.

SELF–HELP PROGRAMME AND LIFESTYLE BALANCE
• Aromatherapy massage for muscle toning.
• Aromatherapy baths.
• Developing a plan to achieve his study and sports goals.
• Learning and using relaxation techniques or meditation for con-centration and sustained energy levels.
• Setting a realistic time schedule to organise all his activities.

SUGGESTED ESSENTIAL OILS
Mental & Emotional Levels:
>Rosemary & Basil for concentration.
>Geranium or Bergamot to refresh him after study periods.
>Frankincense and Rosewood for steady application.
Physical Level:
>Lemongrass & Rosemary in a massage blend applied before and after running.
Suggested Blend:

Rosemary	2
Lemongrass	2
Rosewood	1
	5 drops

Rosemary and Lemongrass are a good combination to help keep Alan's muscles in good condition whilst he is in physical training. Used before running, strains and injuries are less likely. Used after physical exercise they help release muscles and promote better circulation.

Rosemary is a mental stimulant and it is a calming and steadying essential oil. It can help Alan develop the application he will need to discipline himself while preparing for his examinations and the marathon.

8 | Useful Books

Aromatherapy Books

Aromatherapy - A Guide for Home Use	Christine Westwood
Aromatherapy, an A- Z	Patricia Davis
Aromatherapy for Everyone	Robert Tisserand
Aromatherapy for Women	Maggie Tisserand
Encyclopaedia of Essential Oils	Julia Lawless
The Art of Aromatherapy	Robert Tisserand
The Fragrant Pharmacy	Valerie Worwood
The Practice of Aromatherapy	Dr. Jean Valnet

Other Titles

Creating Abundance	Andrew Ferguson
Food and Healing	Anne-Marie Colbin
Games People Play	Eric Berne
Healing Through Touch	John T. Cottingham
I'm OK - You're OK	Thomas A. Harris
Learning to Say No	Carla Wills-Brandon
The Relaxation and Stress Reduction Workbook	Davis, Eshelman, McKay
Stress and Self-Awareness: A Guide for Nurses	Meg Bond
Stress For Success	Dr. Peter Hanson
Understanding Disease	Jon Ball
You Can Heal Your Life & Positive Thinking	Louise L. Hay

9 | Stress Management Essential Oil Guide

Essential oils should always be diluted when used on the skin. Exceptions are Lavender and Tea Tree which may be used neat in the case of burns.

BASIL ~   Key Word: *Clearing*
Latin Name: *Ocimum basilicom*
An excellent aromatic nerve tonic which clears the head and restores strength and clarity to the mind. It is good when sustained concentration is needed (as for exams or driving long distances). Basil essential oil is best administered by a qualified Aromatherapist except for inhalation.

Indications:
Lack of Concentration, Disorganisation, Fainting.

Cautions:
Pregnancy, Sensitive Skin.

BENZOIN ~   Key Word: *Soothing*
Latin Name: *Styrax benzoin*
Benzoin is a warm, soothing and penetrating oil that is good for conditions that are slow to heal. It is particularly excellent for dry cracked skin. Benzoin is a resin and one of the ingredients of "Friar's Balsam".

Indications:
Excessively Demanding, Loneliness, Sadness.

Physical Conditions:
Dry skin.

BERGAMOT ~   Key Word: *Uplifting*
Latin Name: *Citrus bergamia*
Bergamot is valuable for depression and anxiety. It is derived from the rind of a small orange-like fruit native to Italy. Its light, uplifting fragrance blends well with other essential oils.

Indications:
Anxiety, Despondency, Depression, Negative Thoughts, Obsessiveness, Lack of Self-Confidence, Lack of Spontaneity, Staleness, Unco-operativeness.

Cautions:
Do not use within three hours of going in the sun or using a sunbed skin pigmentation may be affected.

BLACK PEPPER ~   Key Word: *Penetrating*
Latin Name: *Piper nigrum*
Black Pepper Oil has a hot, stimulating effect which helps you penetrate the depths of a situation and encourages transformation. It is one of the oldest known spices and was used in India 4,000 years ago.

Indications:
Feeling Powerless or Stuck.

Physical Conditions:
Constipation.

Caution:
Avoid if using homeopathic treatment.

CAJEPUT ~   Key Word: *Focusing*
Latin Name: *Melaleuca leucadendron*
Cajeput is useful because its penetrating aroma helps when you are trying to break old habits and focus on the present.

Indications:
Changeability, Cynicism, Lack of Direction, Disorientation, Inefficiency, Irresponsibility, Procrastination, Lack of Purpose, Lack of Trust, Lack of Understanding, Unreasonableness.

CAMPHOR ~   Key Word: *Piercing*
Latin Name: *Cinnamomum camphora*
Effective when you are suffering from cold, camphor is a powerful oil which also helps you organise your thoughts when your mind is worried and wandering.

Indications:
Avoidance, Lack of Direction, Lack of Perspective, Worry about the Future.

Cautions:
Epilepsy, Homeopathic Treatment, Pregnancy

CARDAMOM ~   Key Word: *Expansion*
Latin Name: Elettaria cardamomum
Cardamom is a good remedy for digestive problems and is a spicy and
warming essential oil. It can help you expand your awareness of internal
problems and help you to be more open.

Indications:
Confusion, Inflexibility, Judgementalness.

CEDARWOOD ~   Key Word: *Steadying*
Latin Name: Juniperus virginiana
Inhaling Cedarwood gives you a steadying effect. It has a long history of
use by the Egyptians and a pleasant smoky odour.

Indications:
Scattered Thoughts

Physical Conditions:
Asthma, Dandruff, Oily Scalp/Skin.

Caution:
Pregnancy

CAMOMILE – MOROCCAN ~
Latin Name: Ormenis multicaulis
References in this book are to Camomile Roman with which Camomile
Moroccan is often confused. This is not a substitute and belongs to a
different plant family.

CAMOMILE – ROMAN ~   Key Word: *Soothing*
Latin Name: Anthemis nobilis
Roman Camomile is one of the most useful essential oils as it is anti-
inflammatory, physically soothing and emotionally calming.

Indications:
Agitation, Lack of Calmness, Over-Excitement, Restlessness, Propensity
to Tantrums, Lack of Tranquillity, Worry.

Physical Conditions:
Bloated Abdomen, Boils, Dermatitis and Other Skin Problems.

CINNAMON BARK ~   Key Word: *Warming*
Latin Name: *Cinnamomun zeylanicum*
Cinnamon bark has traditionally been used as a remedy for digestive problems. It is, however, a powerful skin irritant and should be used with care. It blends well with orange and clove oil in fragrancers but should only be used under guidance of a qualified Aromatherapist for methods other than inhalation.

Indications:
Warming.

Physical Conditions:
Influenza.

Cautions:
Pregnancy, Sensitive Shin

CLARY SAGE ~   Key Word: *Euphoric*
Latin Name: *Salvia sclarea*
Clary Sage is noted for its uplifting effect and warm, nutty scent. It is a good muscle relaxant and a key oil in treatment of Pre-Menstrual Tension.

Indications:
Compulsiveness, Depression, Exhaustion, Listlessness, Nervousness, Obsessiveness, Overly Analytical, Pre-Menstrual Tension.

Caution:
Pregnancy

CLOVE ~   Key Word: *Pain Relieving*
Latin Name: *Eugenia caryophyllata*
Clove is traditionally associated with relief of toothache due to its numbing effect. It is obtained from the flower buds of a small Madagascan evergreen tree and is best administered by a qualified Aromatherapist for uses other than inhalation.

Cautions:
Pregnancy, Sensitive Skin

CORIANDER ~   Key Word: *Motivation*
Latin Name: *Coriandrum sativum*
Coriander is a sweet smelling spicy essence that is stimulating and refreshing in the bath.

Physical Conditions:
Lack of Appetite, Lack of Motivation.

CYPRESS ~   Key Word: *Astringent*
Latin Name: *Cupressus sempervirens*
Cypress's astringent properties make it invaluable for toning. It is
obtained from distillation of the leaves and cones of the Cypress tree
which is native to the Mediterranean.

Indications:
Excessive Talkativeness, Sluggishness.

Physical Conditions:
Asthma, Cellulitis, Dry Ticklish Coughs, Dandruff, Oily Scalp, Heavy
Periods, Excessive Perspiration, Frequent Urination.

EUCALYPTUS ~   Key Word: *Respiratory System*
Latin Name: *Eucalyptus globulus*
Eucalyptus is widely used as an inhalant and chest rub and for its powerful
antiseptic properties. It comes from one of the tallest trees in the world
and exudes an aromatic odour from the entire tree.

Physical Conditions:
Asthma, Colds, Respiratory Tract Infections.

Caution:
Homeopathic Treatment

FENNEL ~   Key Word: *Normalising*
Latin Name: *Foeniculum vulgare*
Fennel is renowned for combating obesity. It was cultivated by the
Romans and was said to convey strength, courage and longevity.

Physical Conditions:
Bloated Abdomen, Excessive Appetite, Indigestion.

Caution:
Pregnancy

FRANKINCENSE ~   Key Word: *Rejuvenating*
Latin Name: *Boswellia thurifera*
Frankincense is extracted from the gum of a small North African tree. It
has a warm spicy scent and has been prized for centuries for skin care and
as an aid to focusing and support in overcoming fevers.

Indications:
Apprehension, Lack of Assertiveness, Lack of Commitment, Lack of
Courage, Lack of Discipline, Doubt, Loss of Faith, Lack of Inner
Strength, Insecure Feelings, Fear of Intimacy, Intimidation, Feeling of
Loss, Lack of Motivation, Nervousness, Nightmares, Over-Cautiousness,
Lack of Perseverance, Possessiveness, Need to be Protected, Feeling
Rejected, Need to be Rejuvenated, Sarcasm, Lack of Security, Lack of
Self-Acceptance, Self-Criticism, Self-Deception, Lack of Self-Worth,
Shame, Lack of Stability, Lack of Stamina, Suspiciousness, Terror, Lack
of Trust, Fear of Unknown Origin, Vulnerability, Lack of Wisdom

Physical Conditions:
Eczema, Scarring.

GERANIUM ~   Key Word: *Balancing*
Latin Name: *Pelargonium odorantissimum*
Geranium is useful for most skin conditions and has a stimulating effect
on the lymphatic system. It blends well with other essential oils and tends
to balance extremes on both the physical and emotional levels.

Indications:
Abrasiveness, Excessive Attachment, Lack of Balance, Emotional
Extremes, Lack of Harmony, Lack of Moderation, Mood Swings, Over-
Powering, Excessive Talkativeness, Lack of Tolerance, Workaholic.

Physical Indications:
Dermatitis, Menopause, Irregular Periods.

GINGER ~   Key Word: *Digestion*
Latin Name: *Zingiber officinale*
Ginger is a warm penetrating oil produced from ginger root by steam
distillation. It should be used in small amounts.

Indications:
Lack of Self-Acceptance, Uncooperativeness.

Physical Conditions:
Colds, Early Stages of Flu.

Caution:
Sensitive Skin

GRAPEFRUIT ~   Keyword: *Releasing*
Latin Name: *Citrus paradisi*
Grapefruit has proved helpful for ditherers and people who are resistant to change. It has a lively, tangy, uplifting aroma.

Indications:
Bitterness, Lack of Clarity, Confusion, Despondency, Envy, Frustration, Lack of Gratitude, Indecisiveness, Meanness, Poor Time Management, Procrastination, Lack of Purpose, Resentment, Self-Pity, Worry about the Past.

JASMINE ~   Key Word: *Expansion*
Latin Name: *Jasminium officinale*
Jasmine promotes emotional openness and sensitivity. Because of its exotic fragrance it is often called the King of the Flower Oils.

Indications:
Doubt of Ability, Apathy, Boredom, Fear of Coming Events, Lack of Communication, Lack of Confidence, Distance, Inability to Express Emotions, Inhibition, Introversion, Jealousy, Judgementalness, Meanness, Over-Analytical, Passivity, Feeling Rejected, Rigidity, Sadness, Secretiveness, Shyness, Lack of Spontaneity, Suppression, Feeling Unloved, Withdrawal.

JUNIPER ~   Key Word: *Purification*
Latin Name: *Juniperus communis*
Juniper essential oil is indicated for its blood purifying and cleansing properties. It is distilled from Juniper berries.

Indications:
Fear of Commitment, Lack of Composure, Laziness, Lethargy, Insensitivity, Lack of Motivation, Over-Sensitivity, Provocativity, Lack of Stamina, Vulnerability.

Physical Conditions:
Cramps, Hangovers, Oedema, Scanty Periods.

Caution:
Pregnancy

LAVENDER ~   Key Word: *Immunity*
Latin Name: *Lavendula officinalis*
Lavender is probably the best-known essential oil and is the Number One choice for the home first-aid kit. It is useful for many physical conditions and helps balance the mind and emotions.

Indications:
Over-Analytical, Anxiety, Fear of Failure, Hyperactivity, Hysteria, Imbalance, Immune System, Impatience, Insecurity, Insomnia, Irrationality, Irritability, Mood Swings, Overwork, Panic, Paranoia, Possessiveness, Greed for Power, Feeling Pressured, Lack of Relaxation, Stage Fright, Tension, Poor Time-Management, Lack of Tolerance, Lack of Tranquillity, Workaholic, Worry.

Physical Conditions:
Baldness, Immune System, Sore Throats, Stiffness, Dermatitis, Eczema, Itchy or Scarred Skin, General First-Aid.

LEMON ~ Key Word: *Refreshing*
Latin Name: *Citrus limonum*
The sharp aroma of Lemon essential oil refreshes and clears the mind. Approximately 3,000 lemons are needed to produce a kilo of the essence, which is made in Sicily from lemon rind.

Indications:
Bewilderment, Complexity, Feeling Misunderstood, Sluggishness, Staleness, Lack of Vitality.

Physical Conditions:
Cellulitis.

LEMONGRASS ~ Key Word: *Strengthening*
Latin Name: *Cymbopogon citratus*
Lemongrass essential oil is derived from a wild grass and is particularly good for the nervous system. It has a powerful attractive aroma that is often compared to lemon sherbet.

Indications:
Boredom, Lack of Concentration, Lack of Creativity, Laziness, Need for Rejuvenation, Sulkiness.

Physical Conditions:
Cramp.

MARJORAM ~ Key Word: *Relaxation*
Latin Name: *Origanum marjorana*
Marjoram promotes deep mental and physical relaxation through its warming qualities and is good for muscle spasm, aches and strains.

Indications:
Hyperactivity, Lack of Moderation, Over-Powering, Lack of Relaxation, Feeling Stuck, Tension.

Physical Conditions:
Cramp.

Caution:
Pregnancy

MELISSA ~   Key Word: *Nurturing*
Latin Name: *Melissa officinalis*
Melissa is a gentle tonic that is useful for allergies. Paracelsus called it the elixir of life. Also known as "Lemon Balm" Melissa encourages feminine qualities such as nurturing and intuition.

Indications:
Addiction, Allergies, Concern, Lack of Humility, Loneliness, Nostalgia, Rejection, Shock, Suspiciousness.

Physical Conditions:
Irregular Periods.

MYRRH ~   Key Word: *Resinous*
Latin Name: *Commiphora myrrha*
Myrrh, which is good for the mouth and throat is, like Frankincense, one of the oldest essential oils and carries religious significance. Ancient Greek soldiers always carried Myrrh with them into battle to treat their wounds.

Physical Conditions:
Dry Coughs.

Caution:
Pregnancy

NEROLI ~   Key Word: *Stress Reliever*
Latin Name: *Citrus bigaradia*
Neroli is the number one oil for stress and shock. It is also known as "Orange Blossom" and has a truly fragrant and settling aroma.

Indications:
Distress, Fear of Future, Hysteria, Feeling of Loss, Overwork, Pessimism, Feelings of Pressure, Restlessness, Shock.

ORANGE ~   Key Word: *Radiance*
Latin Name: *Citrus aurantium*
Orange is a warm cheering oil that is good for sufferers of lethargy or depression.

Indications:
Blaming, Defensiveness, Dullness, Lack of Energy, Hopeless Feelings, Lack of Humour, Negative Thoughts, Over-Controlling Nature, Passivity, Perfectionism, Pessimism, Selfishness, Seriousness, Stubbornness. Sulkiness, Lack of Vitality.

PATCHOULI ~   Key Word: *Penetrating*
Latin Name: *Pogostemon patchouli*
Patchouli is indicated for persistent conditions requiring sustained attention. It is widely used in traditional Indian medicine and has a musky sweet fragrance.

Indications:
Apprehension, Compulsiveness, Greed for Power.

PEPPERMINT ~   Key Word: *Cooling*
Latin Name: *Mentha piperita*
Peppermint is best known as a digestive remedy and a substitute for aspirin. It is cooling on hot summer days when a drop in the bath will leave you feeling refreshed. It is excellent, too, in a foot bath for tired feet.

Indications:
Tardiness.

Physical Conditions:
Aches & Pains, Nausea, Travel Sickness.

PINE (SCOTS) ~   Key Word: *Invigorating*
Latin Name: *Pinus sylvestris*
Scots Pine oil, obtained from pine needles, is a good inhalant and is invigorating in the bath.

Physical Conditions:
Feeling of Weakness, Respiratory Infections.

ROSE OTTO ~   Key Word: *Cleansing*
Latin Name: *Rose centifolia/Rosa damascena*
Rose oil is excellent for physical and emotional cleansing. It acts as a catalyst for change where there are persistent conditions. It is considered to be the Queen of the flowers.

Indications:
Addiction, Allergies, Argumentativeness, Attachment, Bereavement, Clinging, Concern, Dominance, Envy, Grief, Hostility, Insincerity, Nostalgia, Need for Purification, Regretfulness, Rejection, Sadness, Lack of Self-Awareness, Self-Centeredness, Self-Righteousness, Over-Seriousness, Terror, Uncommunicativeness, Unforgivingness, Unhappiness, Fears of Unknown Origin, Feeling Unloved, Unreasonableness, Worry About the Past.

Physical Conditions:
Hangovers.

ROSEMARY ~   Key Word: *Stimulant*
Latin Name: *Rosemarinus officinalis*
A penetrating and stimulating oil which has many mental and physical benefits.

Indications:
Lack of Alertness, Apathy, Boredom, Lack of Clarity, Disorientation, Exhaustion, Fatigue, Forgetfulness, Illogicallity, Indecisiveness, Lethargy, "Monday Morning Feeling", Lack of Motivation, Lack of Objectivity, Poor Time Management, Sarcasm, Sluggishness, Tardiness.

Physical Conditions:
Baldness, Chills, Constipation, Dandruff, Dry Scalp, Cramp, Fainting.

Caution:
Pregnancy

ROSEWOOD ~   Key Word: *Refreshing*
Latin Name: *Aniba rosaeadora*
Rosewood is a pleasant essential oil that has a deep-rooted, steadying effect and boosts creativity.

Indications:
Need for Approval, Challenging, Overly Controlling, Falseness, Feeling Inferior, Paranoia, Perfectionism, Restlessness, Sarcasm, Lack of Stability, Feeling Unappreciated.

41

SAGE ~   Key Word: *Tonic*
Latin Name: *Salvia officinalis*
Sage is an essential oil which is best administered by a qualified Aromatherapist for methods other than inhalation. Its name comes from the Latin for "salvation" and Sage was considered instrumental in the prevention of illness.

Indications:
Lack of Discrimination, Forgetfulness, Erratic Thoughts.

Physical Conditions:
Congestion.

Cautions:
Pregnancy, Sensitive Skin

SANDALWOOD ~   Key Word: *Expression*
Latin Name: *Santalum album*
Sandalwood is traditionally associated with self-expression and is especially useful for throat conditions but is also helpful for the skin. It comes from Mysore in India and has a woody, sweet fragrance.

Indications:
Aggression, Lack of Assertiveness, Clumsiness, Fear of Coming Events, Fear of Conflict, Cynicism, Distress, Fear of Failure, Greed, Lack of Humility, Insensitivity, Lack of Intuition, Listlessness, Lack of Perseverance, Provocativity, Lack of Security, Self-Centeredness, Excessive Self-Criticism, Self-Righteousness, Over-Sensitivity, Lack of Wisdom.

Physical Conditions:
Dry Skin, Dry or Hoarse Throat or Loss of Voice.

TEA TREE ~   Key Word: *Antiseptic*
Latin Name: *Melaleuca alternifolia*
Tea Tree has a strong medicinal smell and has anti-bacterial, anti-viral and anti-fungal effects. It acts as a powerful stimulant to the immune system.

Physical Conditions:
Boils, General First Aid, Respiratory and Throat Infections.

THYME ~   Key Word: *Anti-bacterial*
Latin Name: *Thymus vulgaris*

Thyme essential oil may be freely used in a fragrancer or for inhalations to relieve nasal congestion, but see a qualified Aromatherapist before use in massage or bathing Thyme essential oil is distilled from the flowers of the thyme plant.

Physical Conditions:
Throat and Chest Infections.

YLANG YLANG ~   Key Word: *Confidence*
Latin Name: *Cananga odorata*
Ylang Ylang means "flower of flowers". Its exotic fragrance is warming and helps to instil confidence.

Indications:
Aloofness, Anger, Bossiness, Excessively Demanding, Distance, Guilt, Hostility, Impatience, Introversion, Irrationality, Irresponsibility, Jealousy, Feeling Misunderstood, Over-Analytical Over-Cautiousness, Fear of People, Repression, Resentment, Rigidity, Secretiveness, Lack of Self-Confidence, Lack of Self-Esteem, Lack of Self Worth, Selfishness, Excessive Seriousness, Shame, Shyness, Stage Fright, Stubbornness, Suppression, Withdrawal.

Physical Conditions:
Physical Stress or Palpitations.

10 | Physical Conditions Index

THE SKIN

Affected Area	Method of Use	Essential Oil
Boils	Massage★, Bath, Compress	Camomile
Cellulitis	Massage★, Bath	Cypress, Fennel, Lemon
Dandruff – Dry Scalp	Scalp Treatment	Rosemary
Dandruff – Oily Scalp	Scalp Treatment	Cypress, Cedarwood
Dermatitis	Massage★, Bath, Compress	Camomile, Geranium, Lavender
Dry Skin	Massage★, Bath, Compress	Benzoin, Geranium, Sandalwood
Eczema – Itching or Burning	Massage★, Bath, Compress	Camomile
Eczema – Sensitive	Massage★, Bath, Compress	Geranium & Lavender
Eczema – Skin weeping	Bath, Compress	Lavender & Frankincense
Inflamed Skin	Massage★, Bath, Compress	Camomile
Itchy Skin	Massage★, Bath	Lavender & 1 Drop Peppermint
Perspiration – Excess	Massage★, Bath	Cypress
Pustules	Massage★, Bath, Compress	Tea Tree
Redness	Massage★, Bath, Compress	Camomile
Scarring	Massage★, Bath	Frankincense, Lavender
Skin Type – Dry	Massage★, Bath, Compress	Geranium, Frankincense
Normal	Massage★, Bath, Compress	Geranium
Oily	Massage★, Bath, Compress	Cedarwood, Cypress
Sensitive	Massage★, Bath, Compress	Camomile, Rose

★Massage – *If skin is broken do not massage – Use compress or bathe instead.*

DIGESTIVE AND ELIMINATIVE SYSTEMS

Abdomen Bloated	Massage, Bath, Compress	Camomile, Fennel
Appetite – Excessive	Massage, Bath	Fennel
Appetite – Lack Of	Massage, Bath	Coriander, Rosemary
Constipation	Massage, Bath	Black Pepper, Rosemary
Diarrhoea	Massage, Bath	Black Pepper
Hangover	Massage, Bath	Juniper, Rose
Indigestion	Massage, Bath	Cardamom, Fennel
Headache, Migraine	Bath, Compress, Fragrancer+	Lavender
Travel Sickness, Nausea	Bath, Handkerchief	Peppermint
Urination – Frequent	Massage, Bath	Cypress

RESPIRATORY AND CARDIOVASCULAR SYSTEMS

Affected Area	Method of Use	Essential Oil
Asthma	Massage, Bath, Fragrancer+, Inhalation	Cedarwood, Cypress, Eucalyptus
Coughs	Massage, Bath, Inhalation	Cypress, Sandalwood
Fainting	Inhalation	Basil, Rosemary
Palpitations	Massage, Bath	Ylang Ylang
Voice – Hoarseness	Massage, Bath	Sandalwood

+Fragrancer – *can be used at any time but is particularly beneficial where indicated.*

IMMUNE SYSTEM

Allergies	Massage, Bath	Juniper, Rose
Antibacterial	Massage, Bath, Fragrancer+	Lavender, Tea Tree
Anti-fungal	Massage, Bath	Tea Tree
Anti-viral	Massage, Bath, Fragrancer+	Tea Tree
Colds	Massage, Bath, Fragrancer+	Eucalyptus
Immune System – General	Massage, Bath, Fragrancer+	Lavender, Tea Tree
Influenza	Massage, Bath, Fragrancer+	Cinnamon, Lavender
Oedema	Massage, Bath, Compress	Juniper
Throat – Dry	Massage, Bath	Sandalwood
Infection	Massage, Bath	Tea Tree, Thyme
Sore	Massage, Bath	Lavender, Sandalwood

NERVOUS, HORMONAL AND REPRODUCTIVE SYSTEMS

Adrenal Problems	Massage, Bath	Neroli
Hot Flushes	Massage, Bath	Camomile, Geranium, Melissa
Menopause	Massage, Bath	Geranium
Period – Heavy	Massage, Bath	Cypress
Period – Scanty/Irregular	Massage, Bath	Juniper
PMT† – Tender Breasts	Massage, Bath	Geranium
Water Retention	Massage, Bath	Juniper

†PMT – *Pre-Menstrual Tension*

MUSCULAR, SKELETAL AND CIRCULATORY SYSTEMS

Circulation – Improvement	Massage, Bath	Rosemary
Coldness	Massage, Bath	Rosemary
Cramp	Compress	Juniper
Exhaustion	Massage, Bath	Clary Sage, Lavender
Muscular Aches, Tension	Massage, Bath, Compress	Lemongrass, Rosemary
Stiffness	Massage, Bath	Lavender
Tendons – Over-exertion	Massage, Bath, Compress	Rosemary
Painful	Massage, Bath, Compress	Lavender
Tiredness – Physical	Massage, Bath	Rosemary

11 | Stress Response Index

Response	Change	Essential Oil
Ability – Doubting	Self-Confidence	Jasmine
Abrasiveness	Gentleness	Geranium
Addiction	Freedom	Melissa, Rose
Aggression	Serenity	Sandalwood
Agitation	Serenity	Camomile
Alertness – Lacking	Alertness	Rosemary
Aloofness	Communicativeness	Ylang Ylang
Anger	Forgiving	Ylang Ylang
Anxiety	Optimism	Bergamot, Lavender
Apathy – Emotional/Spiritual	Openness	Jasmine
– Mental/Physical	Enthusiasm	Rosemary
Apprehension	Optimism	Frankincense, Patchouli
Approval – Seeking	Self-Approval	Rosewood
Argumentativeness	Acceptance	Rose
Assertiveness – Lacking	Self-Worth	Frankincense
Attachment	Release	Geranium, Rose
Avoidance	Responsibility	Camphor
Bewilderment	Certainty	Lemon
Bitterness	Gratitude	Grapefruit
Blaming	Acceptance	Orange
Bossiness	Genial Authority	Ylang Ylang
Boredom	Enthusiasm	Lemongrass
Calmness – Lacking	Calmness	Camomile
Challenging	Acceptance	Rosewood
Changeability	Consistency	Cajeput
Clarity – Lacking	Clarity	Grapefruit, Rosemary
Clinging	Releasing	Rose
Clumsiness	Gracefulness	Sandalwood
Commitment – Lacking	Commitment	Frankincense
Complexity	Simplicity	Lemon
Composure – Lacking	Composure	Juniper
Compulsiveness	Freedom	Clary Sage, Patchouli
Concentration – Lacking	Concentration	Basil, Lemongrass
Concern	Acceptance	Melissa, Rose
Confidence – Lacking	Confidence	Jasmine
Conflict	Peace	Sandalwood

Response	Change	Essential Oil
Confusion	Clarity	Cardamom, Grapefruit
Creativity – Lacking	Creativity	Lemongrass
Communication – Lacking	Communicativeness	Jasmine
Courage – Lacking	Courage	Frankincense
Cynicism	Trust	Cajeput, Sandalwood
Defensiveness	Openness	Orange
Dejection	Determination	Bergamot, Frankincense
Demanding	Giving	Benzoin, Ylang Ylang
Depression	Lightness	Bergamot, Clary Sage
Despondency	Upliftment	Bergamot, Grapefruit
Direction – Lacking	Purposefulness	Cajeput, Camphor
Discipline – Lacking	Discipline	Basil, Frankincense
Discrimination – Lacking	Insight	Sage
Dishonesty	Honesty	Frankincense
Disorganisation	Order	Basil
Disorientation	Focus	Cajeput, Rosemary
Distant	Presence	Jasmine, Ylang Ylang
Distracted	Focus	Basil
Distress	Harmony	Neroli, Sandalwood
Dominance	Tenderness	Rose
Doubtful	Faith	Frankincense
Dullness	Alertness	Orange
Emotions – Unexpressed	Openness	Jasmine
– Extremes	Equilibrium	Geranium
Envy	Contentment	Grapefruit, Rose
Exhaustion	Vigour	Basil, Rosemary
Erratic Thoughts	Focus	Sage
Faith – Loss Of	Faith	Frankincense
Falseness	Self-Acceptance	Rosewood
Fatigue	Energy	Rosemary
Fear – Of Commitment	Responsibility	Juniper
– Of Conflict	Peace	Sandalwood
– Of Coming Events	Adventurousness	Jasmine, Sandalwood
– Of Failure	Confidence	Lavender, Sandalwood
– Of People	Gregariousness	Ylang Ylang
– Of Unknown Origin	Trust	Frankincense, Rose
Feeling – Hopeless	Optimism	Orange
– Inferior	Self-Regard	Rosewood
– Insecure	Security	Frankincense
– Intimidated	Assertiveness	Frankincense
– Loss	Comfort	Neroli
– Misunderstood	Clarity	Lemon, Ylang Ylang
– Powerless	Empowerment	Black Pepper
– Pressured	Relaxation	Lavender

Response	Change	Essential Oil
Feeling – Rejection	Self-Appreciation	Melissa, Rose
– Stuck	Transformation	Marjoram, Black Pepper
– Unappreciated	Self-Appreciation	Rosewood
– Unloved	Loving	Rose, Jasmine
– Weak	Strength	Pine
Forgetfulness	Mindfulness	Sage
Frustration	Appreciation	Grapefruit
Gratitude – Lacking	Gratitude	Grapefruit
Greed – For Possessions	Generosity	Sandalwood
– For Power	Fulfilment	Lavender, Patchouli
Grief	Acceptance	Rose
Guilt	Self-Forgiveness	Ylang Ylang
Hesitancy	Adventurousness	Jasmine
Hostility	Warmth	Rose, Ylang Ylang
Humility – Lacking	Humility	Melissa, Sandalwood
Humour – Lacking	Humour	Orange
Hysteria	Composure	Neroli, Lavender
Hyperactivity	Steadiness	Lavender, Marjoram
Illogicality	Logicality	Rosemary
Indecisiveness	Decisiveness	Grapefruit, Rosemary
Impatience	Patience	Lavender, Ylang Ylang
Inattentiveness	Attentiveness	Rosemary
Inefficiency	Efficiency	Cajeput
Inflexibility	Flexibility	Cardamom
Inharmonious	Harmoniousness	Geranium
Inhibition	Expressiveness	Jasmine
Insomnia	Repose	Lavender
Insecurity	Security	Frankincense, Lavender
Insensitivity	Sensitivity	Juniper, Sandalwood
Insincerity	Sincerity	Rose
Intuition – Lacking	Intuition	Sandalwood
Irrationality	Rationality	Lavender, Ylang Ylang
Irresponsibility	Responsibility	Cajeput, Ylang Ylang
Irritability	Calmness	Lavender
Introversion	Gregariousness	Jasmine, Ylang Ylang
Jealously	Generosity	Jasmine, Ylang Ylang
Judgementalness	Acceptance	Cardamom, Jasmine
Laziness	Vigour	Lemongrass, Juniper
Lethargy	Vivacity	Juniper, Rosemary
Listlessness	Stability	Clary Sage, Sandalwood
Loneliness	Self-Appreciation	Benzoin, Melissa
Loss	Acceptance	Frankincense, Neroli
Meanness	Generosity	Grapefruit, Jasmine
Moderation – Lacking	Moderation	Geranium, Marjoram

Response	Change	Essential Oil
Monday Morning Feeling	Enthusiasm	Rosemary & Citrus Oils
Mood Swings	Stability	Geranium, Lavender
Motivation – Lacking	Motivation	Coriander
Negative Thoughts	Positivity	Bergamot, Orange
Nervousness	Ease	Clary Sage, Frankincense
Nightmares	Peace	Frankincense
Nostalgia	Presence	Melissa, Rose
Obsessiveness	Flexibility	Bergamot, Clary Sage, Lavender
Over-Analytical	Intuition	Clary Sage, Jasmine
Over-Cautious	Confidence	Frankincense, Ylang Ylang
Over-Controlling	Relaxation	Orange, Rosewood
Over-Excitement	Poise	Camomile
Over-Powering	Moderation	Geranium, Marjoram
Over-Sensitivity	Objectivity	Juniper, Sandalwood
Overwork	Steadiness	Lavender, Neroli
Panic	Calmness	Lavender
Paranoia	Trust	Lavender, Rosewood
Passivity	Vivacity	Jasmine, Orange
Perfectionism	Pragmatism	Orange
Perseverance – Lacking	Perseverance	Frankincense, Sandalwood
Perspective – Lacking	Perspective	Cardamom, Camphor
Pessimism	Optimism	Orange, Neroli
Possessiveness	Generosity	Frankincense, Lavender
Purpose – Lacking	Purposefulness	Cajeput, Grapefruit
Procrastination	Efficiency	Cajeput, Grapefruit
Protection – Need For	Courageousness	Frankincense
Purification – Need For	Purification	Rose
Rejuvenation – Need For	Vitality	Frankincense, Lemongrass
Regretful	Acceptance	Rose
Relaxation – Lacking	Relaxation	Lavender, Marjoram
Restlessness	Equilibrium	Camomile, Neroli, Rosewood
Repression	Expressiveness	Jasmine, Ylang Ylang
Resentment	Forgiveness	Grapefruit, Ylang Ylang
Rigidity	Flexibility	Jasmine, Ylang Ylang
Sadness	Joyfulness	Benzoin, Jasmine, Rose
Sarcasm	Supportiveness	Frankincense, Rosewood
Scattered Thoughts	Composure	Cedarwood
Security – Lacking	Feeling Secure	Frankincense, Sandalwood
Secretiveness	Openness	Jasmine, Ylang Ylang
Self-Acceptance – Lacking	Self-Acceptance	Ginger, Frankincense
Self-Awareness – Lacking	Self-Awareness	Rose
Self-Centeredness	Involvement	Rose, Sandalwood
Self-Confidence – Lacking	Self-Confidence	Bergamot, Ylang Ylang
Self-Critical	Self-Approval	Frankincense, Sandalwood

Response	Change	Essential Oil
Self-Esteem – Lacking	Self-Esteem	Ylang Ylang
Self-Pity	Self-Appreciation	Grapefruit
Self-Righteousness	Humility	Rose, Sandalwood
Self-Worth – Lacking	Self-Worth	Frankincense, Ylang Ylang
Selfishness	Unselfishness	Orange, Ylang Ylang
Seriousness	Humourousness	Orange, Rose, Ylang Ylang
Shame	Self-Respect	Frankincense, Ylang Ylang
Shock	Peace	Melissa, Neroli
Shyness	Naturalness	Jasmine, Ylang Ylang
Sluggishness	Vigour	Cypress, Lemon, Rosemary
Spontaneity – Lacking	Spontaneity	Bergamot, Jasmine
Stability – Lacking	Stability	Frankincense, Rosewood
Stage Fright	Self-Confidence	Lavender, Ylang Ylang
Staleness	Enthusiasm	Bergamot, Lemon
Stamina – Lacking	Strength	Frankincense, Juniper
Stubbornness	Willingness	Orange, Ylang Ylang
Sulkiness	Cheerfulness	Lemongrass, Orange
Suppression	Expression	Jasmine, Ylang Ylang
Suspiciousness	Discernment	Frankincense, Melissa
Talkative Excessive	Receptivity	Cypress, Geranium
Tantrums	Equanimity	Camomile
Tardiness	Promptness	Peppermint, Rosemary
Tension	Relaxation	Lavender, Marjoram
Terror	Calmness	Frankincense, Rose
Tolerance – Lacking	Tolerance	Geranium, Lavender
Tranquillity – Lacking	Tranquillity	Camomile, Lavender
Trust – Lacking	Trust	Cajeput, Frankincense
Unbalanced	Balance	Geranium, Lavender
Uncommunicative	Communicativity	Jasmine, Rose
Uncooperative	Cooperativeness	Bergamot, Ginger
Understanding – Lacking	Insight	Cajeput
Unforgiving	Forgiving	Rose
Unhappy	Happiness	Jasmine, Rose
Unmotivated	Motivation	Juniper, Rosemary
Unreasonable	Considerate	Cajeput, Rose
Vitality – Lacking	Vitality	Lemon, Orange
Vulnerability	Empowerment	Frankincense, Juniper
Wisdom – Lacking	Wisdom	Frankincense, Sandalwood
Withdrawn	Affectionate	Jasmine, Ylang Ylang
Workaholic	Harmony, Steadiness Perspective	Geranium, Lavender, Marjoram
Worry – General	Stability	Camomile, Lavender
Worry – About Future	Trust	Camphor, Melissa, Sandalwood
Worry – About Past	Presence	Grapefruit, Rose